The Live Lean Detox Plan

Five days step by step vitality plan

Chantal Di Donato

Live Lean Health Ltd.

DEDICATION

This plan is dedicated to you, wonderful women and men, who are ready to start living your most authentic health ever. In today's messy world, with so much poison in our food, we just don't know how we should really feel anymore. We may take a pill when we have a headache, stomach ache, digestive issues or feel pain, but how about giving our body the tools it needs to heal itself? You need to start somewhere, and this is the first step, a five days guided plan to help you strengthen your body's natural detoxifying skin

CONTENTS

ACKNOWLEDGMENTS

This guide and its content are not meant to substitute for medical care. The content is educational and informative for leading a healthy lifestyle. If under medical care and taking medication, you should consult your physician in relations to changes in your diet.

INTRODUCTION

The Live Lean Detox Plan, is a 5 days guide to expel toxins from your body effortlessly. The human body is a perfect creation, it can heal itself given a chance.

Here is yours; to start this wonderful journey without any long term commitment. Before going ahead , it is clear to understand that this plan is not a diet. We are all different and the way we should eat varies between person to person, but we all need to cleanse our system every now and then. For more information about bio-individuality please speak to us and visit our website, www.liveleanhealth.com , as a follow up to this five days plan.

Why is the Live Lean Detox different?

Most detox programs entail some sort of limitation in food intake and cause feeling hungry and drowsy. Our plan is to make you feel amazing in just 5 days by eating whole foods, which not only stimulate your system and help it detoxify, but also nourish you completely. No need to take pills or buy expensive products, you just need to follow the plan, invest in natural and organic foods and let your body do its job.

What side effects can be expected?

As you rid your body of toxins, gluten, sugars, dairy and caffeine, you may experience a slight headache for the first couple of days of the program. This is a normal reaction and it will go away. Drinking plenty of water and herbal tea, to stay hydrated and aid detoxification, will decrease the side effects you may be experiencing.

What is the key component to the Live Lean Detox Plan?

The Plan is completely vegan. A diet with no animal products and focused mainly on phytochemicals, vitamins, antioxidants, natural fats and fiber, will help your whole system heal. For some of us, a diet without meat can seem a challenge, but don't worry, once you have cleansed your system, you can start implementing your favorite meat and dairy into your diet. The only difference will be, you will feel so much better and know what source of animal protein works best for you.

What results should be expected?

In a nutshell, you will feel amazing after only 5 days. Some of the benefits of this program are:
 More energy
 Feel leaner and lighter
 Fewer aches and pains
 Deeper quality sleep
 Better bowel movement
 Stronger immune system
 Better mood
 Shinier hair
 Clearer skin
 Clearer eyes
 Overall wellness
 A continuous sensation of
 unprecedented wellbeing

And the list continues. If you suffer from ailments such as Candidiasis[1], you will also find that your symptoms will get better because you are nourishing your system with probiotics rich foods and powerful phytochemicals which starve the yeast.

---

[1] Candidiasis: Yeast Infection affecting particularly women. It can cause vaginal discharges and lower immune system when the yeast grows within our digestive system, mainly the gut.

LET'S GET STARTED

Before getting into the five days detox plan, there are a 5 steps to take, in order to make this experience enjoyable and worth your effort and time.

1. Start stocking your home with the foods you should be eating for the next five days. At the end of this booklet, we have created a shopping list for you, to make this process easier.

2. Buy a diary and record your progress and feelings everyday. This is particularly important when you have completed the five days detox and are implementing other foods into your diet.

3. Keep a positive mindset by starting your morning with positive affirmations. This will allow you to cleanse your body with the foods advised, but also your mind.

4. Enjoy the process. If you love food, then enjoy your daily intake of the best, most real food you can possibly find. Those foods can be easily incorporated into your lifestyle after the cleanse and actually should

5. Be open mind about this experience. There might be foods you may have not experimented with before, like superfoods into your smoothies or juices. Be open minded about this experience and try to see what you like and what you can substitute.

DAY 1

Drink 2 liters of water and herbal teas per day (no sugar or milk added)

Breakfast

Start your morning with a large glass of water and 1 spoon of unpasteurized Apple Cider Vinegar.

Super smoothie

- 50% baby spinach
- 1 stalk celery
- 1 spoon freshly squeezed lemon juice
- Pinch of cayenne pepper
- 1 tsp. **Organic Detox mix**[2]

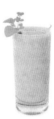

---

[2] The inSpiral Detox Mix is a great combination of wheatgrass, spirulina, milk thistle, barleygrass, chlorella and zeolite powder. You can opt for those ingredients singularly, as they are sold separately as well.

Depending on your lifestyle you could add more food to your breakfast:

Simple Oats

- Uncontaminated oats (gluten free)
- 1 spoon of chia seeds
- 1 tsp. of raw honey (Please note that if you have infections, or cancer, you should avoid sweeteners)
  Boil water and add to the oats and chia seeds. Let it cook for 4 minutes. Add the raw honey and enjoy.

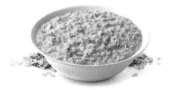

Morning Snack

Despite controversial opinions on snacking, I personally believe it can be extremely beneficial if done well. What I mean by that is that I see it as an opportunity to add more nutrients to our diet and help the body detoxify.

Nori vegetable wrap

As an alternative to wheat, Nori is not only easy to prepare, but extremely healthy. Seaweed is full of protein and great source of iodine, which

promotes a healthy thyroid function.
- 2 x nori sheets
- 1 spoon of hummus (please buy organic, or home made)[3]
- Rocket salad
- Sprouts of choice

Spread the hummus on the nori sheet. Leave 50mm on the side empty. Add rocket and sprouts and roll the nori sheets and enjoy the 2 wonderfully healthy rolls.

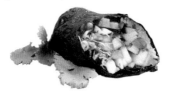

Lunch

Quinoa Warm Vegetable Salad

- Cooked quinoa, warm or cold
- Roasted root vegetables (cooked in coconut or olive oil) with rosemary and sea salt (or Himalayan)
- Boiled green beans
- Garlic
- Chillies
- Ginger

---

[3] Home made hummous: cooked chickpeas, spoon of tahini, 1 tsp. lemon juice, salt and olive oil – blend together

Mix all the ingredients and add fresh extra virgin olive oil (1 spoon) and enjoy this satiating meal which contains great protein , fatty acids and phytochemicals. Your body will love it

Afternoon Snack

Booster smoothie / Juice

- Broccoli
- Ginger
- Lemon
- Celery
- 1 tsp.. **Vitality Mix**[4]

This extremely detoxing blend, will stop your sugar cravings and give you all the energy needed to perform for the rest of the afternoon. Cleansing and detoxifying is about giving the body energy to get rid of the toxins, so this will do the trick.

---

[4] inSpiral vitality mix is a great blend of: maca, yacon, baobab, reishi extract, ginseng, acai and purple corn

Dinner
Rawlicious salad

Going to bed feeling light is so important. We do not want to burden the body with heavy foods to digest when we want to make sure the energy used by the body goes towards repairing tissues and getting rid of the toxins within our system by stimulating our colon, so that we can expel waste first thing in the morning (after our tall glass of water with apple cider vinegar)

- Romaine lettuce
- ½ cucumber
- ½ yellow pepper
- 1 asparagus
- 1 carrot
- Avocado
- Goji berries
- Cabbage
- Olive oil
- Sea or Himalayan salt
- Apple cider vinegar or lemon

Chop all ingredients finely and toss them together with olive oil, salt and apple cider vinegar or lemon.

Due to the cooling effects of the raw vegetables, if you feel cold or unsatisfied, feel free to have a cup of miso soup. Buy fermented brown nice and soy miso paste and add to water after it has boiled, not to kill the probiotics within the miso, as it is a fermented food.

First night detox ritual

To allow your body to start detoxifying, the first day will end with taking 1 active charcoal tablet before bed. Please do not take the tablet with your food or with any vitamins. Charcoal attracts metals, toxins, any compound found on its way through the GI. It is therefore very important to not eat food as nutrients won't be assimilated by the body. So wait 2 hours after supper to take it. Drink 1 pint of water with it, as it can be quite dehydrating; it may cause thirst during the night

DAY 2

Drink 2 liters of water and herbal teas per day (no sugar or milk added)

Breakfast

Start your morning with a large glass of water and 1 spoon of unpasteurized Apple Cider Vinegar.

Anti inflammatory mix

While detoxifying, we are focusing on making our body more alkaline so to stop inflammation. Toxins cause inflammation which in turn, can cause many of the ailments we face today, including cancer.

- 1 celery stalk
- 1 bunch of fresh parsley
- Blueberries
- 1 spoon lime
- 1 spoon lemon
- Flax seeds
- 1 tsp. **Organic Detox mix**

Depending on your lifestyle you could add more food to your breakfast:

Super Chia starter

- 2 spoons Chia seeds
- Coconut shreds (unsweetened)
- Almond milk (unsweetened)

Mix together In a blender till the mixture becomes quite thick like a pudding. Sprinkle some Goji berries on top and enjoy.

Morning Snack

Coconut kefir and strawberries

- Organic and unsweetened coconut kefir
- Organic Strawberries (or other berries)

Lunch

Lentils soup

- Lentils (soaked for at least 12 hours if dry. If using canned lentils, please make sure they are preserved in water only.
- 2 fresh tomatoes
- 2 spoons olive oil
- Garlic
- Oregano
- Parsley

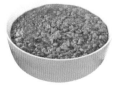

Mix all the ingredients and cook for 1 ½ hours. Add water if it starts becoming dry; you need to keep this quite liquid in order to aid digestion. As a side dish, prepare a small, simple salad:

- Arugula
- Avocado
- Flax seeds
- Sour kraut (organic)
- Olive Oil
- Sea or Himalayan salt

Afternoon Snack

Cancer fighting smoothie / Juice

- Romaine lettuce
- ½ pineapple
- ½ banana
- ½ cup blueberries
- 1 Spoon raw, unsweetened cacao

Tip: did you know? Raw cacao is the most powerful antioxidant on the planet?

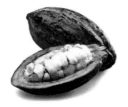

Dinner

Super Carrot soup

- 3 carrots
- 1 bunch of coriander
- Organic vegetable stock (low sodium)
- Mixed seeds

Chop the carrots finely and boil in water for 20 minutes until soft but still have a crunch. Add the carrots broth to a glass blender and add vegetable stock to the boiling water. Add coriander and blend together. Once smooth, sprinkle with mixed seeds.

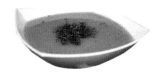

DAY 3

Drink 2 liters of water and herbal teas per day
(no sugar or milk added)

Breakfast

Start your morning with a large glass of water
and 1 spoon of unpasteurized Apple Cider
Vinegar.

Bowel regulator smoothie

- 1 handful kale
- ½ beetroot
- ½ apple
- 1 spoon lemon
- Cold herbal tea /water or coconut
  water
- 1 tsp. **Organic Detox mix**

Mid morning snack:

Carrots with aubergine dip

A great way to have complex carbohydrates
(from vegetables) and protein, allowing the body
to digest and detox easily

- 2 peeled carrots (to eat raw)

Dip:
- 1 aubergine (roasted in the oven and cooled)
- 1 spoon of tahini
- Pinch of sea or Himalayan salt
- 1 spoon olive oil
- 1 tsp. lemon juice
- ½ clove of garlic

Place the aubergine in a blender with or without skin, as you prefer. Mix all the ingredients in the blender until it is creamy and enjoy with the raw carrots

Lunch:

Chickpeas salad

- ½ cup of chickpeas (you can either use water canned or prepare the chickpeas making sure you soak them in water for at least 12 hours and after rinsing, leave them to soak with bicarbonate of soda for 1 hours before cooking. Rinse them well before cooking and boil them for 2 hours with garlic and olive oil
- Roasted butternut
- Rocket and watercress leaves
- Fresh tomatoes

- Olive oil
- Sea or Himalayan salt
- Sesame seeds

After having prepared the chick peas (prepare the day before or when you have time; they can be stored well in the fridge) and roasted the butternut, mix all other fresh ingredients and add chickpeas and butternut. Mix well with olive oil and salt and sprinkle with sesame seeds

TIP: boil the butternut prior to roasting.

Afternoon Snack

- 1 cup of blueberries
- Herbal tea

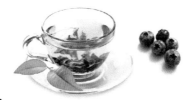

Dinner

Tomatoes and corgettes salad

- 8 Fresh tomatoes
- 2 courgettes
- Garlic
- Oregano
- Coriander
- Toasted seeds

- Goji berries
- Olive oil
- Sea or Himalayan salt

Blend the tomatoes with water to liquefy and have a soupy consistency.

Chop the courgettes in very small cubes

Pre heat olive oil in the pan with garlic and add the courgettes until soft

Add the rest of the ingredients and let cook for 20 minutes

Add toasted seeds on top and enjoy!

DAY 4

Drink 2 liters of water and herbal teas per day (no sugar or milk added)

Breakfast

Start your morning with a large glass of water and 1 spoon of unpasteurized Apple Cider Vinegar.

Wake up blast

- 1 celery stick
- Arugula
- 1 orange
- 1 spoon lemon
- Cold green tea
- 1 tbs **Organic Detox mix**

Morning snack

Quinoa wrap

- 2 Nori sheets
- Organic or home made plain hummus
- ½ avocado
- Quinoa
- Sprouts

Spread the hummus on to the Nori sheets , add

the sprouts, quinoa and avocado and roll. Enjoy them and their detoxing power

Lunch

Kelp spaghetti blast

-   Kelp spaghetti (Available from Planet Organic or Whole Foods)
-   ½ red sweet pepper
-   ½ yellow sweet pepper
-   Cucumber
-   Kale
-   Chilli flakes
-   Garlic
-   Olive oil
-   Sea and Himalayan salt

Rinse the kelp spaghetti with warm water. Chop all the vegetables in small cubes , add them to the Kelp, add olive oil and salt and toss well before enjoying a great detoxing dish.

Tip: sprinkle some green Nori sprinkle.

Afternoon snack

Super veggie power

-   Handful of baby spinach
-   1 small head of broccoli
-   1 celery stick

- 2 pineapple rings
- Green tea
- 1 tsp.. **Vitality mix**

Dinner

Pea, pumpkin creamy soup and brown rice

- 1 cup of small peas
- 2 cups chopped pumpkin
- ½ red onion
- 1 clove of garlic
- Lemongrass
- Pinch of grated ginger
- Chopped parsley
- Sea or Himalaya salt
- Brown jasmine rice
- Olive oil

Boil the rice separately until cooked and let it set.
Chop onion, garlic, ginger and parsley and mix together in the pot with olive oil. Let it sizzle until slightly golden.
Add peas and pumpkin into the mix and stir fry slightly, add 4 cups of water and the rest of the ingredients. Let it boil for 1 hours and keep it liquid. Once cooked, blend the mix and make it creamy, then pour over some rice and enjoy.

Tip: Sprinkle some roasted coconut shreds for a great oriental flavor with the lemon grass.

DAY 5

Drink 2 liters of water and herbal teas per day (no sugar or milk added)

Breakfast

Start your morning with a large glass of water and 1 spoon of unpasteurized Apple Cider Vinegar.

Wake me up before you detox smoothie

- 1 cup beetroot juice (freshly pressed)
- 2 celery sticks
- 2 pineapple rings
- Pinch of cayenne pepper
- Ice green tea (home made the night before)
- 1 tsp.. **Organic Detox mix**

Blend all the ingredients and add the cayenne pepper on top.

Morning snack

Goji mix

- Handful of mixed raw seeds
- Handful of organic Goji berries

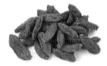

Lunch

Magic Quinoa soup

- Cooked quinoa
- 3 carrots
- 1 broccoli bunch
- Paprika
- Ginger
- 1 spoon raw honey
- Olive oil
- Sea or Himalayan salt
- Garlic
- Coriander

Boil the quinoa separately. Chop the carrots and broccoli. Pan fry garlic, ginger and olive oil. Add the vegetables with ½ pot of water and add in the coriander and paprika. Boil for 30 minutes and see if the vegetables are cooked to your liking but still have a crunch. Once cooked, blend the mixture if you like (optional you can keep the vegetables chunk, if you cut them small) and add a spoon of honey and 2 spoons of quinoa to the mix.

Tip: add more water if you don't want this too creamy

Afternoon snack

Hormones boost (smooth juice)

- ½ cup beetroot juice (freshly pressed)
- ½ cup broccoli and kale juice (freshly pressed)
- 10 raspberries
- 10 blueberries
- ½ avocado
- 25 ml of Aloe Vera[5]
- 1 tsp. probiotic powder

Add the fresh juices to the solid ingredients to smooth together.

---

[5] Aloe Vera is a powerful detoxifier, please do not use if pregnant and do not feed to infants and small children.

Dinner

Half rawlicious last supper

- Kelp noodles
- 1/2 tbs coconut oil
- 3 stalks small broccoli
- 6 broad beans
- ½ cup shredded red cabbage
- 6 organic tomatoes
- 1 shallot
- Sea or Himalayan salt
- Cayenne pepper

Soak kelp noodles in warm water for 3 minutes. Meanwhile shred the shallot and pan fry lightly with the coconut oil. Chop and shred all other vegetables and cook lightly, they need to be crunchy. Once done, add the drained kelp noodles and mix together.

Bon Apetit!

FOLLOW UP

Before starting your Live Lean Detox plan, you may be afraid that you will be hungry through this process, and as a result, miserable. But I have designed this plan keeping in mind you need energy for your daily chores an activities and I wanted to make detox an easy process. You may be a big meat eater and being on a vegan detox may be too much for you.

The reality is that the body can only detox with the help of a plant based diet because phytochemicals, which nourish, support and stimulate our cells, are only found in living foods, such as vegetables.

But what this 5 days plan will do for you, is create an energy and purity never felt before. The good news? After only 5 days you will see some drastic changes in your skin, hair, water retention, digestion and overall energy levels.

The way this plan is designed will allow you to incorporate one detox day a week even when you go back to eating the way you did before, if you wish.

What I do recommend, is that you keep juicing and smoothing your vegetables and fruit, particularly if you are not big on eating raw vegetables.

Extra tips that you can implement into your detox and as a follow up are:

- Take 25ml Aloe Vera juice daily for a month[6]. It will help digestion and cleanse your colon daily, reflecting on your skin. You will literally GLOW!
- Take good quality and powerful strain of probiotics daily. Probiotics heal the gut and keep us regular. Expelling toxins via our digestive tract stimulates a strong immune system and prevents severe illnesses.
- Drink enough water per day. Though 2 liters is standard, you may be very active and need more, so listen to your body beyond the recommended quantity.
- Take care of yourself: detoxing internally is key, but we are exposed to environmental toxins which our skin protects us from, but is inevitably affected by. The tips below can help you detox on the outside as well and feel and look better:
  - Face scrub daily naturally. Mix

---

[6] Aloe Vera is a powerful detoxifier, please do not use if pregnant and do not feed to infants and small children.

finely ground oatmeal with coconut oil and scrub your skin thoroughly. Rinse well and add moisturize

- Would you like to have a natural moisturizer too? Save a 20ml bottle and fill ½ way with grapeseed oil and ¾ with almond oil. Add 10 drops each of 100% pure essential oils: lavender, ylang ylang and bergamot. (For oily skin add tea tree instead of ylang ylang). Cheaper and more natural than any other moisturizer.

- Scrub your body weekly. This is one of the uses for sugar, I am not opposed to. Mix coarse brown sugar with 100% lemongrass and lavender essential oils and coconut or almond oil. Store in a glass jar for multiple usage and scrub once a week on dry skin. Rinse off and enjoy a wonderfully radiant and smooth skin.

- Massage your body and take care of it. Coconut oil, Cacao butter, almond, grape seeds, jojoba or avocado oils are great for moisturizing the skin and replenishing it.

- Take care of your back. Our backs suffer constantly from standing, seating in font of computers, carrying heavy weights and not always having the right posture. At Live Lean we work with Ayurvedic oils, especially designed to reduce pain in the back in a completely natural way and more effectively than commercial gels.

- Do Yoga and feel the difference. Yoga is a very powerful practice for your body and your mind. It can detoxify both by allowing you to realign your energy and connect your thoughts to your actions. You do not need to be flexible and experienced. All that matters is the time you dedicate to yourself during practice and you will see your progress once you are committed to it.
- Disconnect and distress by taking some time out. Did you know that stress is one of the worst toxins for your body? Even if 30 minutes a day, take time to do nothing and completely let go of chores, responsibilities and worries. This will allow your body to built strength and regulate your hormones, which will help detoxify, together with good nutrition.
- Implement good habits into your lifestyle, past the 5 days plan. Aside from juicing, use superfoods daily as part of your nutritional plan and let it do the magic. The detox and vitality powders are a great way to add superfoods to your fresh juices and smoothies daily. You will love them.

This plan and the extra tips given have been written with love. I want you to experience energy, vitality and health everyday, for the rest of your life. We take our health for granted until it is gone, and we should preserve it because it is the only asset which is really ours. Be willing to commit the time to cook, prepare and eat fresh foods and invest in yourself as the rewards will be off the charts.

ABOUT LIVE LEAN

Live Lean Health was born last November, after years of studying and learning by its founder Chantal Di Donato. Live Lean focuses on helping women balance their hormones for better skin, weight loss, fatigue control, immunity boosting and overall wellness. It also helps women go through healthy pregnancies by preparing the body for this wonderful 9 months long journey through to how to feel and look amazing post partum. Hormones control everything in our bodies. Visit our website for more information
www.liveleanhealth.com

ABOUT CHANTAL

Chantal is a Certified Holistic Health Coach and founder of Live Lean Health. She graduated from the Institute of Integrative Nutrition (IIN) in NYC, and undergoing her Yoga training at Aditya Yoga School. Her journey started 16 years ago after two years long battle with anorexia and 15 years destructive relationship with food. She turned her life around and is now focusing on helping others find balance. Author of the Live Lean Health Plan and creator of the Live Lean inspirational Cards, a set of beautiful images and words to help create daily positive intentions. Find more about her websites or email Chantal@liveleanhealth.com

DETOX SHOPPING LIST

This shopping list will help you plan for your 5 days detox by stocking all the relevant ingredients to your daily meals. I have listed them as they appear per day with the exception of duplicates. Most ingredients can be purchased at health stores such as Whole Foods and Planet Organic and the superfoods powder can be purchased with us directly.

Baby spinach
Organic celery
Lemon
Cayenne pepper
Organic Detox Mix* [7]
Uncontaminated gluten
free oats
Raw honey
Nori Sheets
Organic plain hummus
Rocket
Sprouts
Quinoa
Pumpkin
Sweet potato
Parnsnip
Green beans
Garlic
Chillies
Ginger
Pure sea or Himalayan salt
Broccoli

---

[7] * inSpiral Organic Detox mix included is part of this Detox plan package. For more you can purchase it on our website www.liveleanhealth.com

Organic Vitality mix *[8]
Broccoli
Romaine lettuce
Cucumber
Peppers (red and yellow)
Asparagus
Carrots
Avocado
Goji berries
Cabbage (red and white)
Extra virgin olive oil
Coconut oil
Lime
Blueberries
Flax seeds
Chia seeds
Mixed seeds
Shredded coconut
Unsweetened almond milk
Lentils
Tomatoes
Oregano
Parsley
Pineapple
Banana
Apple
Cacao
Coriander
Vegetables stock
Arugula
Sour kraut
Herbal teas (of choice)
Green tea
Coconut water

---

[8] You can purchase this from our website:
www.liveleanhealth.com

(unsweetened)
Beetroot
Aubergines
Kale
Tahini
Chickpeas
Watercress
Sesame seeds
Courgettes
Kelp spaghetti
Peas
Red onion
Lemongrass
Brown jasmine or basmati
rice
Paprika
Raspberries
Broad beans
Shallot
Aloe Vera liquid*[9]
**Multibillion acidophilus
(probiotics)*[10]**

---

[9] You can buy the Aloe Vera liquid in any health stores in their holistic therapy department

[10] You can buy probiotics in any health stores or pharmacy